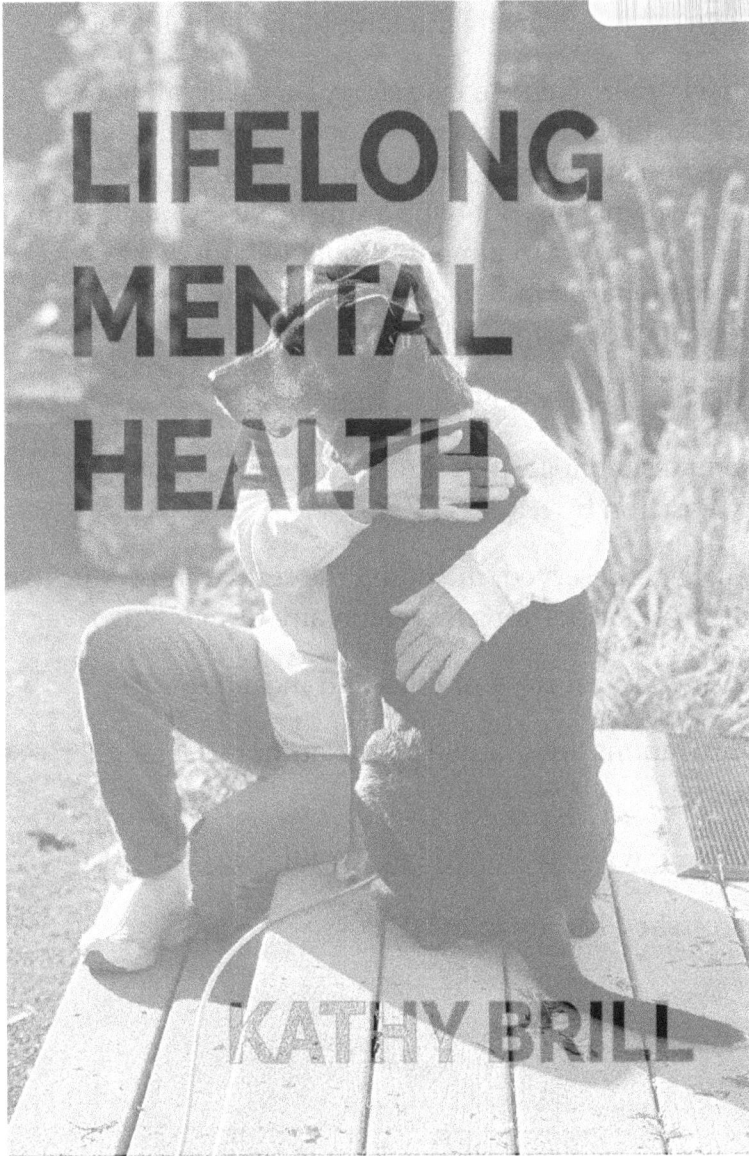

LIFELONG MENTAL HEALTH

KATHY BRILL

Dedication

To my mother as forgiveness for not realizing how important she was to her children.

To my husband and two daughters. Without all of you, life would not have been worth living. You have repeatedly helped me realize how important I am in your lives.

The darkness of mental illness is not a friend. There are no clear-cut edges, just an infinite heavy feeling shoving patients in all directions.

This is one patient's true story about the involuntary control mental illness can have over patients. No hope for a cure. No end in sight. Just constant pressure turning conscious thought into chaos.

Patients are not doomed to this torturous life. Good quality of life IS possible despite a diagnosis. This patient's story is proof.

TABLE OF CONTENTS

PROLOGUE

How much can one person really be expected to take? Nothing about living life is easy, even for those deemed psychologically and physically balanced and healthy. A person trying to survive in today's challenging society needs every edge possible. A supportive circle of people who give a darn is at the top of that needs list (Li et al, 2021). Now insert a mental illness diagnosis into that picture. The 'needs list' just changed drastically.

What defines life as good? This is a true story about one patient, Eliza, sharing her lifelong struggle to live a good life despite her diagnosis. Through each battle between her mind and life's challenges, she fought to land back on her feet. Eliza's medical diagnosis of clinical depression and anxiety finally came at age 47. Up until that point, Eliza felt like an outcast, not fitting in with peers or as a new employee on the job. All through her life Eliza continually tried to educate family and friends about her illness so they could provide the support she needed. She sought answers from medical professionals about living with the daily psychological challenges. She learned that medication is not enough.

This is Eliza's rollercoaster ride through life with a mental illness. What is written between these pages are Eliza's thoughts and feelings. This story is told through the patient's lens. Eliza's character and personality were built from her experiences around people and places. Her mind compartmentalized these experiences by how they left her feeling – upset, afraid, nervous, embarrassed, humiliated, sad, happy, etc. As Eliza passed through each phase of her life, these compartments continually expanded to make room for each new set of circumstances. Eliza believes this flexibility was key to not only allow her to survive but to ultimately thrive!

Readers are invited to join Eliza on her rollercoaster ride through life with a mental illness, to hear her voice and learn from her survival strategies during the most torturous times. May Eliza's strong will to keep on living serve as inspiration, education and hope for anyone struggling to live with a mental illness.

PHASE ONE – EXCLUSIVE RIDE TIME

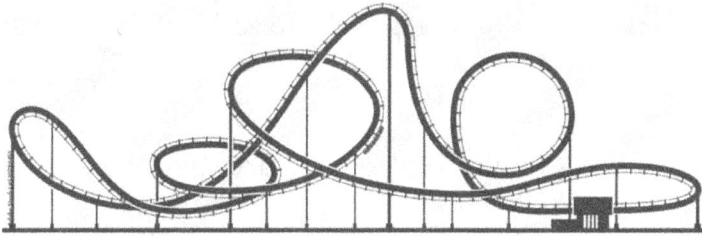

This is Eliza's exclusive ride time (ERT) (Helbig, 2022) on life's mental illness rollercoaster. There are no other members of the ERT club on board. There's one slippery bench for Eliza to sit on, equipped with a headrest and individual lap bar (Helbig, 2022). She has no idea when the ride will start or what to expect after it begins. There are no instructions provided and only a marginal presence by family and a few friends as she zooms past them. Eliza didn't have a say about whether she would like to take the ride. She was just suddenly plopped down on the bench.

BIRTH TO AGE 10 – DIVING RIGHT IN

Eliza was born on Tuesday, June 17, 1958, weighing 6.5 pounds. She was born into a mixed ethnicity home. They were a family unit of six, first two boys then, a dozen years later, two girls, with Eliza being the youngest. Their names are Blake, David, Sarah and Eliza.

Eliza's first home was a small three-bedroom home in Levittown, Pennsylvania. Eliza shared her bedroom with her sister, Sarah, who was two years older. Her older brothers, Blake and David, shared the other bedroom, while Mother and Father sometimes slept together in the master bedroom. Fights between Eliza's parents happened several times a week often leaving one of them sleeping on the sofa.

This first family home was sparsely furnished with secondhand furniture. The window treatments consisted of miscellaneous random large pieces of cloth loosely tacked up above the windows. The house was surrounded by a small plot of grass. There was a rusted chain-link fence enclosing the back yard with a small concrete patio.

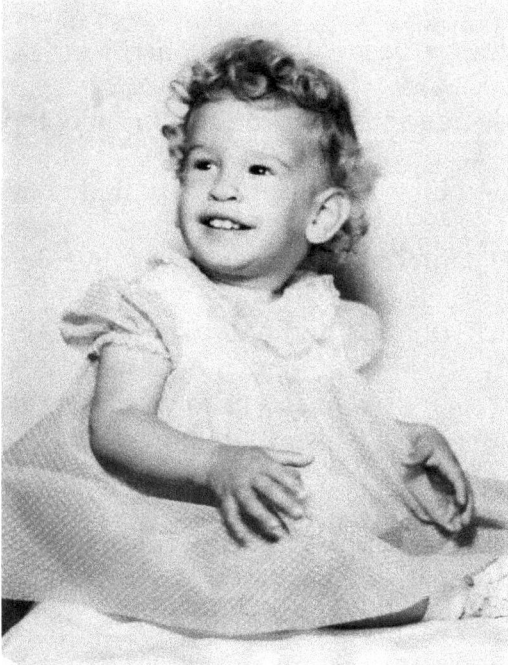

Young Eliza

Eliza was the youngest child in the community. Eliza lived a quiet, solitary life and found solace by playing with her dolls and giving them her unlimited love. She would put herself down for a nap with her dolls in most any place in the house. Once, at age 3, Eliza decided to nap on the metal tray under their outside barbecue. The entire house, a group of neighbors and local law enforcement searched for hours trying to find her in the community. Before darkness hit, Eliza was spotted on a tray under the barbecue. Everyone had a great laugh as her Father decided it would be fun to videotape her as Mother tapped Eliza to wake up. Eliza had no idea there was such a panicked search. She just wanted a nap. Looking back on this today as an adult, Eliza was surprised so many people went to great lengths to find her.

One day the community kids decided to let Eliza join their play sessions. Eliza was so happy to be included in the group. She soon realized the invitation was all one-sided when the kids told Eliza they were going to play football and required Eliza's head be the football! It was either that or go back home alone. Eliza dutifully ran around with her head clutched in the crook of someone's arm. She endured several play dates doing this until the older kids just lost interest. Being the youngest in the neighborhood, Eliza wasn't able to find her own friends.

One evening Sarah was having trouble understanding her homework. Mother sat at the table trying to tutor her but quickly ran out of patience and slapped Sarah's forehead causing her head to bend backwards. Sarah's tears had no impact on Mother. Sarah's punishing session sitting next to Mother trying to comprehend the homework continued until bedtime. Eliza sat quietly at the end of the table waiting to go to bed with her sister. This was the first time Eliza witnessed a beating.

Blake and David were high school age and got into mischief as much as possible. In the early 1960s, youths often drank alcohol during social gatherings. Blake was the popular one with David in his shadow. Misadventure often started by Blake losing his temper and saying whatever he liked without concern for consequence, just like Father.

"Child maltreatment is a devastating type of adverse childhood experience that encompasses neglect and emotional, physical, and sexual abuse (including sex trafficking). Adverse childhood experiences are exposures to maltreatment or household dysfunction during crucial developmental periods that disrupt neurodevelopment and can result in lifelong physical and psychological harm, altering the child's behavior and disease risk into adulthood."

(Suniega et al, 2022)

Many a time the brothers came in late causing Mother a great deal of worry. When Father decided he heard enough of Mother's crying, he quickly lashed out at the boys when they returned home one evening. There was a good deal of yelling and backtalk. It was not uncommon for Father to fling Blake down on the sofa and choke him until he apologized. The turbulent time all parents go through when their children are teenagers was handled in Eliza's home with yelling, physical pinning down and painful pressure applied until her brothers surrendered. Eliza was always present at home and within listening range. She was too terrified to come out of her room to watch. Isolation was her only comfort. On more than one occasion, the police were called, and Father was locked up for the night.

The family relocated often, going from one small town and state to another. No reason was ever given to the children about why so much moving around, leaving no time for family home memories to form. Every house was plain and ordinary, furnished with secondhand furniture and just enough food to survive. Mother made the girls' clothes by hand. There were no family dinners. Eliza's home was filled with yelling, hitting and neglect.

A leather belt hung on the dining room wall as a reminder of the consequence of lying, about anything at all. When the belt was not easily handy, a switch was cut from long thin branches in the brush around the house.

It felt like a whip. The girls were hit just enough to sting and leave red marks, but no bruises to show proof. With the brothers, dad did not hesitate to put his hands around their neck. The girls lived in fear of the next beating. No hugs goodnight or wishes for sweet dreams from the parents ever. No reading aloud or spending time with the children. The children just tried to stay out of the way and go unnoticed.

At age 5, with no explanation given to the Eliza or Sarah, the parents decided to move to Smyrna, Delaware. They rented an old farmhouse that seemed huge to Eliza. There was a lot more room there than she had ever seen before. The girls had their own playroom with a very old homemade television. Watching television was only allowed when the children happened to be in that room playing at the same time Mother or Father wanted to watch a show. There was a twin bed in this room, one upholstered chair, their toybox and enough floor space for imaginary doll play.

Eliza's solace was playing alone for many hours in the playroom with her dolls. She used books propped up on end as walls for the rooms in the doll house. Eliza felt spooked going upstairs alone in the big farmhouse. She spent a lot of time at the foot of the stairs looking up longingly.

Eliza went to kindergarten at Clayton Elementary School. She was so frightened on her first day, she peed down her legs while standing in line with the other children. Feeling ashamed, Eliza kept her head bowed.

> "Shame represents a painful emotion that implies a devaluation of the entire self and dispositional inadequacy, often making the individual feel as if he/she was naked and exposed to others' judgement."
>
> (Maggi et al, 2022)

The fear soon subsided when a cute boy named Randy befriended Eliza in first grade. They often played the 'penny game' where Randy would push a penny up through a crack in his wooden desk and Eliza would try to grab it. This happened almost every morning before classes began. Unbeknownst to Eliza, Randy secretly wanted to give Eliza her first kiss. Randy attempted this in the cloak room just outside the classroom. Things happened quickly and soon became clumsy. Randy's first and only kiss landed right on Eliza's eyelid.

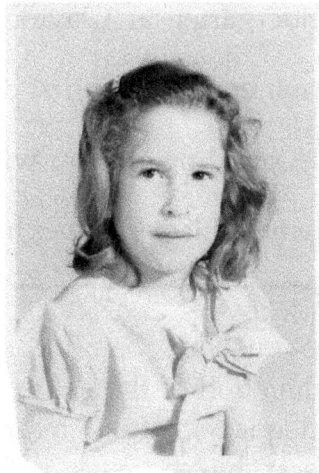

Eliza - First Grade

Both Blake and David found odd jobs in the small town of Smyrna until the Vietnam war draft came up. Blake enlisted in the Army and, soon after, David was drafted into the Marines. Eliza remembers Mother being very upset about David being on the front line of war.

There was concern that David may never make it back home.

Sarah and Eliza were often left alone to entertain themselves. They were sent outside to play and be out of the way. Sometimes goofy mischief prevailed and one of them would go crying to Mother who immediately demanded to know whose fault it was. Neither Sarah or Eliza would agree on the answer, so Mother resorted to taking the belt off the wall and giving them both a bare bottom beating. These types of beating scenes happened several times a week and often with very little provocation. Eliza remembers admitting lying to Mother about brushing her teeth. The punishment for this little fib was another belt beating.

Sarah and Eliza rarely were invited to ride in the backseat of their Ford Studebaker when her parent's wanted to have a family outing. It never took long for Sarah and Eliza to start goofing around and being loud. When Mother decided it needed to stop, she would suddenly turn around and slap both girls across the face with one full swing. The girls sat quietly for the rest of the trip.

At age 6 Eliza witnessed her Mother's seizure for the first time. The seizures started happening a few years earlier. Now Eliza was old enough to remember the frightening scene of Father trying to put a ruler in her mouth to prevent tongue swallowing and the ambulance sirens rushing away to the hospital with her Mother. Mother's seizures were mostly mild and could be contained if Eliza and Sarah (at the young ages of 5 and 7) saw the seizure coming and could get Mother to swallow her medication, Dilantin. The diagnosis was a brain tumor that continued to grow with each year. Mother refused surgery because, back in 1965, the procedures were invasive and required head shaving.

Mother's tumor had grown so large that Mother spent most days laying down feeling severe pressure and headaches. In 1968 surgery was attempted to save her life, but the surgeon told Father the tumor had spread too much. One evening Father put both Sarah and Eliza on his lap on the chair in the playroom and told them, "God took mommy." On February 9, 1968, Eliza's Mother died. The first thought Eliza had in her head was "good, no more beatings." Eliza was nine years old.

A funeral was held at the local Methodist church in town. All members of the extended family came out of the woodwork to attend the gathering at the farmhouse. This was the first time Eliza met many of them. Several women from the community and church handled cooking the food and cleaning up. Both brothers were granted military leave to attend. The next day everyone left, and the house was empty and silent.

Eliza and her sister, ages 9 and 11, were now 'latchkey kids', fending independently for themselves both before and after school. Father didn't walk outside and wait with them for the bus like Mother used to do.

Nor was he home to receive them off the school bus. Father spent little time with the girls and had no idea what was needed to take proper care of them. Come that summer, with no discussion ahead of time, Father shipped Sarah and Eliza off to aunt's and uncle's houses until the next school year began. That was the end of the family farmhouse.

By age 10, Eliza independently developed her first coping skills:

- Isolation in her bedroom or the playroom alone with her dolls and away from her parent's emotional zone,

- Speaking very little and making minimal eye contact to avoid assumptions about her thoughts,

- Seldom asking questions or making a request for anything, even for a simple ice cream cone,

- Not entering her parent's bedroom or Father's office under any circumstance, and

- Always being obedient and honest to avoid scolding.

DISCUSSION

The foundation of a child's life begins at home. Children are at the mercy of everyone around them. They are born innocent and molded a little bit every day by the actions of others. What a parent does and how they do it is a model for their children. The same applies to older siblings and other family members that spend a good bit of time with those children.

A child is born into a prearranged living situation. How that child copes, who provides love and guidance, and where each choice takes them is rarely within their control. Eliza learned through instinct how to live well through sheer survival instincts and a strong will.

It is said that people are a result of their upbringing (Barchi, 2024), and sometimes the luck of the draw. (Merriam-Webster, n.d.). The people involved in a person's life are as important as the roof over their head. People learn from each other every day, be it through online platforms or direct one-on-one encounters. Every situation presents a choice. A person who was not surrounded and guided by good people as they grew up is ill-equipped to make the best choice.

Children are more observant than parents realize. They have a keen sense of the body language around them. Every household has a unique dynamic between its inhabitants which grows and changes over time. Early in life, a child becomes a part of that dynamic and contributes to it, even if they are too young to walk and talk (Syakhrani et al, 2024).

Eliza instinctively knew what she needed to do when she was afraid. A child's "fight or flight" response (Chu et al, 2024) isn't a decision; rather they are only equipped to run away from the fear source. It's interesting Eliza chose to nap under the barbecue; why not nap in her room?

> "**A stressful situation,** whether environmental or psychological, can activate a cascade of stress hormones that produce physiological changes. Activating the sympathetic nervous system in this manner triggers an acute stress response called the **fight**-or-**flight** response. This response enables an individual to either fight the threat or flee the situation. The net effect allows a person to perform more strenuous activity than usual. After the perceived threat disappears, their body return to basal levels."
>
> (Chu et al, 2024)

Routines help children feel safe (Syakhrani et al, 2024). School days should be consistently similar. Responsible adults or family should see their children off to school and welcome then back home afterwards. A wonderful bonus is to ask children, "how was your day?" Children under the age of 12 should not be left alone to fend for themselves (Sultana et al, 2024). They need someone to make sure breakfast is eaten, lunch is provided, and dinner is routinely held with the family unit together. Children need their guardian to help with homework, wash their clothes, make sure personal hygiene is covered and, for goodness' sake, someone to say "goodnight." Eliza had none of these things.

The Beauty of Routines

- "Definition of child routines – regular, repetitive behaviors involving a child and an adult. This includes both child- and caregiver-initiated routines, covering activities like bedtime, mealtime, and chores."
- "The establishment of routines in families tends to foster elevated self-confidence, self-esteem, and self-reliance in children and adolescents."
- "Home routines positively influence a child's school experience and academic outcomes by aiding adaptation to school routines and enhancing cognitive development, self-regulation, and language skills."

(Selman et al, 2023)

PHASE TWO – TWISTED

Eliza had no idea what the future held for her. To survive she had to adjust to an empty house with no adult guidance or support. Eliza endured fierce school bullying in grades eight and nine. No adults helped Eliza comprehend and handle all the psychological and physical challenges her body would soon go through. Eliza felt most helpless during these years, sometimes twisted tight and other times unraveled and falling apart.

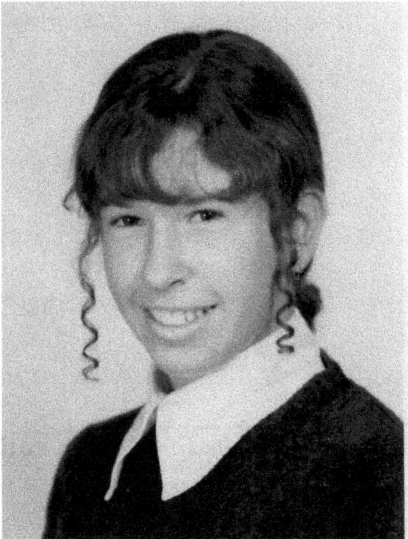

Eliza age 11

AGE 10 TO 18 – FIRST STEPS TOWARD

INDEPENDENCE

Eliza attended public school for grades six and seven. Sarah and Eliza were well-behaved latch-key kids. Father went out every Saturday night and left the girls alone all night. They didn't know how to cook meals and mainly lived off hot dogs, French fries and baked beans. Their brother, David, gave his sisters a mini lesson in how to fry eggs. Eliza's first try at making something completely on her own was a failure; she made potato salad but didn't know to cook the potatoes first. David and Sarah reminded her of this funny mistake often.

By age 13, Eliza seemed to be finished growing, settling in at a height of 60 inches. Her hair was dark brown, very curly and often frizzy. She didn't have access to hair products or any idea how to use them. As soon as her hair was long enough, Eliza braided it every day to keep it under control. Her complexion was fair, taking after her Mother's Irish side of the family.

Sarah was the mischievous one climbing out her bedroom window and going off in a car with her boyfriend who was years older. One Saturday evening, Sarah decided the boys should come to our home and that they did. Everyone except Eliza drank and smoked cigarettes. That night Father suddenly came home, and the boys went running out the back door. Father confiscated all the alcohol and tobacco and locked it in the kitchen china cabinet for his daughters to look at every day. No beating, just psychological shaming.

Starting in grade seven, Father decided Sarah and Eliza would be better placed in a Catholic School. Eliza's class was broken into two distinctions, those we received high grades and those who did not. Eliza was in the 'not so brilliant class.' One boy, Mark, often sat behind Eliza and amused himself by squirting glue in her hair. Fortunately, Mark was the only annoying boy in her class. Eliza only saw her best friend, Patti, during recess because she was in the 'brilliant class.'

A few years later, Father suddenly decided he no longer wanted to be responsible for Eliza and Sarah, so they were sent to live with their older brother, Blake, in Pennsylvania. Blake was married with two young children and lived in a two-bedroom apartment. Eliza and Sarah shared a bedroom with Blake's daughter, Tina. It was crowded but clean and decently furnished.

Blake inherited his Father's short temper. Eliza witnessed one beating of Tina. Blake lost his temper over something trivial when Tina froze with fear and would not answer his question. Tina had only her panties on at the time. Blake pulled them off and put Tina over his knee for a bare bottom spanking. Tina was so terrified she peed all over her Father's legs. Eliza remembers Blake laughing about that while Tina ran back into her bedroom. Blake continued to physically abuse Tina until he went too far and social services took her out of the home.

Eliza's eighth and ninth grade school years were the most torturous. Eliza had no choice but to ride the school bus. She endured having food and trash thrown at her during the entire journey with cruel, cutting remarks. Some mornings Eliza really wanted to just walk away when the school bus came. She didn't because she knew in her heart it was the wrong thing to do. Even if Eliza did have the courage to walk away from the bus, there was nowhere else for her to be that day. Going back to Blake's apartment was not an option. There were no friends or other adults to help. No one listened to Eliza.

Bullying

- Bullying is a form of violence, inflicting profound psychological impact, especially on adolescents.
- Violence from bullying is an *intentional* behavior characterized physical assault and mental stress. No one bullies by mistake.
- This trauma could lead to the death or disability of the victim, and may also cause serious consequences in family and social relationships.

(Huang, 2023)

Once during Social Studies class, Eliza was so upset about the ride into school, she lowered her head and held it in her hands at her desk. She welled up and tried not to cry. Everything in the classroom was quiet because students were just given a reading assignment. Upon looking up for a second, Eliza found the teacher's eyes focused on her. She quickly returned to the assignment to avoid any questions. The teacher never pulled her aside and did not refer her to the school counselor. If only the teacher had done *something*.

At age 16, Eliza felt uncomfortable living in cramped quarters with Blake and his family. Their home was not a happy one. In addition, Eliza really had enough of bullying from peers.

Eliza requested a move to her Father's home in Delaware with the hope of making new friends and enjoying more of life. It was just Eliza and her Father living in a small ranch home. Father worked every day and spent most evenings hanging out at the local VFW bar. Every Saturday, Father spent all night out dancing and drinking. This is the time when Eliza learned to cook proper meals for herself. Eliza drove herself to school and private piano lessons. She was studious, getting top grades in her class. Eliza spent most of her time alone at home studying or playing classical piano, four to six hours a day. She felt lonely and believed she was not pretty. There were no boyfriends at the time. Looking back now, Eliza realized there were a couple of admirers, but she didn't recognize the flirting. Girlfriends were few and not to be counted on during rough times. She felt a heavy weight went with her everywhere. She had no tools or advice to teach her how understand these feelings.

In her junior year of high school, Eliza was diagnosed with trichomonas vaginalis, a sexually transmitted disease. At her first gynecologic exam, she told the doctor, "That is impossible because I am a virgin." The doctor then suggested perhaps she contracted it off a public toilet seat. From there Eliza was sent to another gynecologist and was told it was necessary to have a procedure called cervical cryosurgery. With no mother or other woman to advise Eliza at that time, she dutifully followed the physician's instructions. The procedure was explained to Eliza, but the possible consequences were not. The trichomonas *was* cured but the hymen covering the vaginal opening was broken, making it seem like she was not a virgin to her first partner. This left Eliza feeling ashamed.

Eliza missed a week of high school because of dental surgery. No note was sent to the school because Father never paid attention to those details and Eliza didn't know a note was needed. Upon returning to school, the high school counselor called her to the office to inquire why she hadn't been at school. After Eliza explained, the counselor accepted the reason as acceptable but requested that it not happen again. Eliza responded, "I didn't think you cared." Looking back now, Eliza realizes they didn't care but were instead thinking of truancy. No high school counseling was ever encouraged for Eliza and was never initiated by counselors unless to confirm acceptable absence. It's as if she were present for class but absent to the school staff.

Eliza's first real job was at age 16 as a maid in her uncle's motel in Wildwood, New Jersey. There she felt loved and cared for by her aunt and uncle. They always made her feel welcome. Not once did they raise their voices. Eliza earned enough money to start her first bank account and independently bought all her school supplies for the next year.

At age 17, Eliza felt pushed by her Father to excel in playing classical piano. Her Father decided this was her best possible vocation and felt free to tell everyone. Eliza scored extremely low on her SAT exams and was refused admittance to college. Eliza's brother, David, told her, "Your school has let you down." Eliza believed her high school counselors failed to do their job of advising Eliza about how to best prepare for the SATs. Feeling very low self-esteem, Eliza decided to back away from the pressure of everything and gave up piano. This was met with yelling and shaming of Eliza by her Father. Father was angry Eliza had stopped playing piano and took every opportunity to let her know his disappointment. There were no discussions with Father; one did as he dictated or left.

At the close of Eliza's senior year, the English teacher assigned students to read *Brothers Karamazov* and to come to the final class prepared to write an essay. Eliza opened the book many times but could not get through the reading. During the essay period in class, Eliza wrote a note to the teacher telling her she felt overwhelmed with sadness and loneliness at home and asked for her forgiveness. Eliza graduated high school at age 18, coming down from an A grade to a C grade in English. She was full of self-doubt and believed she really didn't have any particular talent.

Eliza independently found a full-time job in the mailroom of the Dupont company in Wilmington, Delaware. She commuted two hours each workday riding public transportation. She often spent evenings alone at her Father's home in Delaware. Friends were hard to come by and never visited.

Things became strained between Eliza and Father after she started dating. Once Father sat in his recliner while Eliza waited for her date to arrive. He repeatedly scoffed, "he probably isn't going to show up, you know!" Her date did in fact show up and Eliza returned several hours later to a dark, quiet house. Soon thereafter, Eliza and her Father refused to speak to each other.

Eliza found an unfurnished apartment close to work and soon moved out with her personal things loaded in her car. Upon learning this, Father immediately took the car keys away from Eliza, leaving her with nothing but public transportation to get to work and the grocery store. Eliza slept on the floor of her first apartment using some of her clothes as a cushion. She hand-washed her clothes in the bathtub and strewed them out on the apartment floor to dry. With minimal income, Eliza ate very little food and felt weak. The only highlight in her life happened when a friend came and picked her up occasionally on the weekend to get out and have fun.

It wasn't until Eliza became an adult that she learned both her parents had a mental illness. Back then in the 1950's, mental health diagnosis and treatment seldom happened. Both brothers suffered from Vietnam War post-traumatic stress disorder (PTSD). Her sister was the only one in their family unit of six to be spared mental illness. Learning of the family inheritance of mental illness helped Eliza understand a little more about

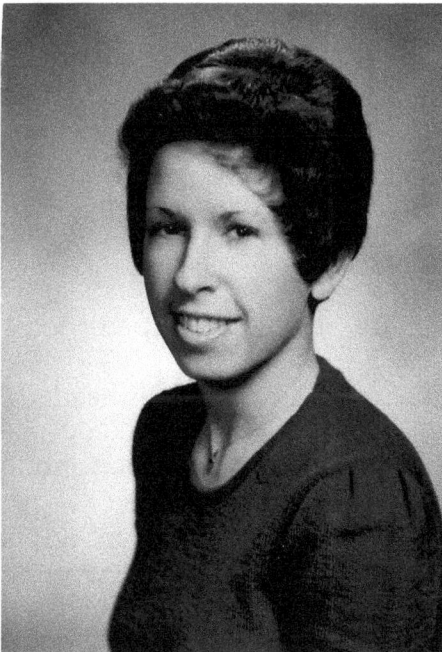

Eliza age 18

herself.

By age 18, Eliza adapted and expanded her coping skills:

- Meditation through hours of focused classical piano playing,

- Focused learning: books often opened on the table partnered with a pencil and notebook,

- Watching television, usually alone in Father's living room,

- Minimal socialization with peers, preferring introverted activities, and

- Seldom leaving the house.

DISCUSSION

Teenagers are as unequipped to handle the psychological and physical changes headed their way as newborns. Puberty has been described as one of the most "profound biological transitions in a person's life" (Susman and Rogol, 2014). Teenagers need help understanding their rapid physical changes but, more importantly, understanding their social and emotional development. "The prefrontal cortex is one of the last regions of the brain to reach maturation, which explains why some adolescents exhibit behavioral immaturity. The fact that brain development is not complete until near the age of 25 years refers specifically to the development of the prefrontal cortex" (Arain et al, 2013). A parent or guardian has the weighted responsibility to walk that teenage path with their children. Without that support, it would be akin to leaving your child completely alone and vulnerable to many evil things in society.

Puberty is characterized by both physical and neurological changes (Best and Ban, 2021). A flux of hormonal activity has been linked to changes in behavior. Recent research suggests the brain is not just developing but changing during this period, with a remodeling of the prefrontal cortex of the brain. This part of a young person's brain involves decision-making and is directly related to the planning and understanding of their actions (Choudhury et al, 2008).

The basic common sense of knowing right from wrong is not yet present in a teenage brain. Consequences of their actions can be life changing and forever scarring. Just one wrong choice, being in the wrong place at the wrong time, very easily pulls a child down a dangerous path. The hardest part of parenting is knowing that your child is making poor decisions and having absolutely no control over their very active social schedule. Now flip that around to the hardest part of being a child or teenager – when there are no responsible, trusted adults to lean on for guidance.

All of these new-fangled electronic connections and apps have created a disconnected society. There is unbridled freedom to search for anyone anywhere around the world through just a few keystrokes. Misplaced keystrokes present huge risks to privacy for everyone. Our disconnected society has become an individualistic nightmare, with profound impact on the mental health of today's youth and young adults (Wickramaratne et al, 2022). These are the crucial years for cognitive development and, without connectedness with someone trusted, where is there to turn for insight, answers, best next steps?

PHASE THREE – STEEP CLIMB

The next eight years of Eliza's life would be her poorest and loneliest. This period of her life would reveal the coldness of her family and the tremendous challenge of trying to live independently. With each year that passed, life's ladder got tougher financially and psychologically. Eliza made repeated attempts to reposition her ladder or move it to a completely different spot to get the best possible footing toward happiness and financial comfort.

AGE 18 TO 26 – NO TURNING BACK

At age 19, Eliza decided to quit her job and move to Virginia to be closer to her brother, David. Her total belongings were packed into her car. Eliza easily found a job and a furnished trailer to rent. Her salary was just at minimal wage, leaving Eliza struggling to make ends meet.

During her stay in Virginia, Eliza fell deeply in love but was not loved in return. Breaking up with her love was the hardest thing Eliza ever did, leaving her with a broken heart and gut-wrenching anguish. This sad time was topped off with her car engine failing, leaving Eliza totally stranded with no public transportation.

To improve her life, Eliza reached out to her sister and brother-in-law in New Jersey. They offered her a bedroom for temporary stay. Eliza left behind anything that didn't fit into a car, leaving furniture she was still paying for and her unrepairable car. She rented a car and drove to New Jersey.

Soon after moving in with them, Eliza felt unwelcome to eat their food, use their laundry facilities and even be present in the same room with them. After only a few months, Eliza was asked to leave by her sister. Eliza got a job and bought a used car to be independent. She worked two jobs to make ends meet and lived alone in sparsely furnished garage apartment near to both jobs. This lasted less than a year because Eliza again reached the point of complete exhaustion. Good roommates were impossible to find, and Eliza still didn't have any good friends.

Eliza really needed to make a change for the better. She was welcomed into the home of a distant friend in Elkton, Maryland. Her friend, John, and his Mother were so kind and accepted $25 a week for rent. This arrangement worked for a short time until John decided he would like to have on-demand sex with Eliza. No love; just lust. He was very pushy.

Searching for a way out, Eliza once again found an inexpensive apartment in a building surrounded by elderly tenants and owned by a very kind landlord. She had to start working two jobs again to pay the bills. Here she stayed until a wonderful bright light finally shone in her direction.

The last attempt toward independence, at age 26 changed Eliza's life forever. Her best friend, Patti, from eighth grade, played matchmaker and arranged for a blind date. Six weeks later Eliza became engaged. She and her fiancé wed three months later, and Eliza never looked back.

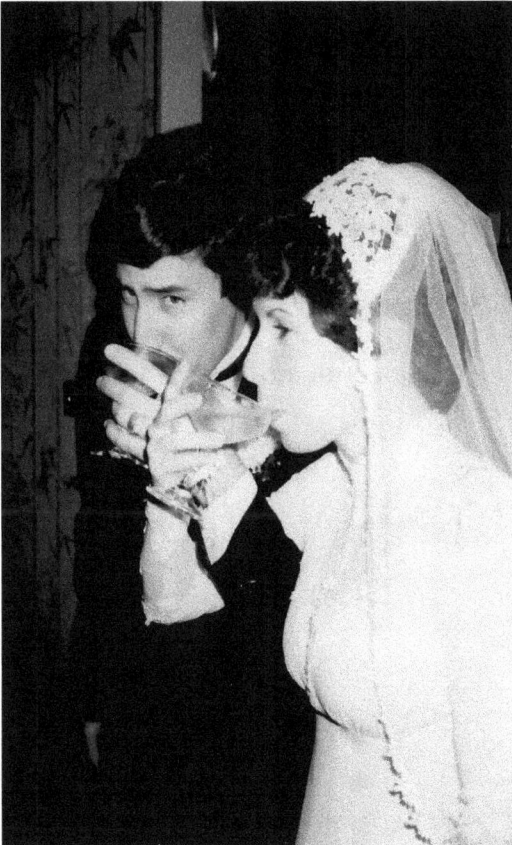

Newlyweds wedding toast

By age 26, Eliza fine-tuned and expanded her coping skills to distract her from feeling completely alone and exhausted from overwork:

- Working two jobs to eliminate financial stress,

- Borrow the use of a piano after her second job shift was over at a nursing facility, as Eliza no longer had her own piano to use,

- Exercising as much as possible,

- Focusing on part-time college courses at the University of Delaware,

- Seldom socializing, with no true friends in the area and a dislike for alcohol and drugs,

- Spending leisure time laying on her bed listening to the radio and daydreaming of better times to come.

DISCUSSION

This span of Eliza's life was spent learning right from wrong and dealing with the consequences of her decisions. Eliza had several failed attempts to be a successful, independent woman. There were no opportunities to put life in reverse and try a different path. Each journey toward independence took time until failure was realized, taking a little bit of Eliza's resilience away. Each new attempt felt less exciting and much more formidable because the odds of success were not in Eliza's favor. The roads all seemed to lead to the same place. The motor was still running but the wheels were just spinning in place. Eliza gradually collected lessons learned from her failures – deciding who is trustworthy, realizing how important her car is to independence, and accepting that she may never be free from working two jobs.

Not an optimistic future for Eliza's crystal ball for sure. There is something to be said for the character traits of stubbornness and a strong will. It remains a puzzle to even the most brilliant medical and scientific minds how a person can overcome impossible circumstances in life and just keep plugging along. Eliza was repeatedly defeated but certainly not dissuaded from trying again. People can learn, adjust, reassess and persevere more robustly than any computer. There's no "blue screen of death" (Hristova, 2017) for people who are stuck. There may be momentary silence while the human mind is clearing "cache" and sorting through erroneous information. A solution is either reached or the goal is changed to compensate for outliers. People are the most complex processing organisms on earth. Add to that a mental illness diagnosis and these people almost become wonders of nature, repeatedly fighting through a web of darkness littered with obstacles, only to come out repeatedly on top.

PHASE FOUR – NEW POINT OF VIEW

Eliza embarked on a brand-new journey with her new husband and his family. She was expected to be wife and daughter-in-law now. Eliza was born with an independent mind and fierce determination to reach her goals. She would not be controlled or told *how* to feel. She also would not be called a "housewife." Eliza earned an income and lived under the same roof as her husband's family, but continued to do some of her favorite things separate from them. The next nine years were a dual track journey for Eliza.

AGE 26 TO 35 – FRESH START

Eliza's wedding dress was borrowed from her sister and the event had less than fifty friends and family in attendance. It was a rainy day, which many said is good luck. Eliza ignored negative comments from family and co-workers. She knew in her heart this was a good decision. Eliza made many adjustments from living alone independently to now living with her new husband and his family. Eliza selflessly offered to move in with his family to reduce disruption to her new family and promote a smooth transition to married life.

They were happily married. Eliza's best friend, Patti, commented that it was impossible to get a molecule of air between them! Their weekly activity included attending a concert at the Academy of Music in Philadelphia every Saturday evening. Eliza's husband generously gave her the cash to have their family piano refurbished. Eliza now once again enjoyed playing classical music. Early in the marriage, there was little talk about starting their own family unit together. When Eliza did bring up the subject, her husband made it very clear he didn't want anything to do with babies and dirty diapers. Eliza listened but did not comment; rather, she kept her secret wish to create her own family unit one day with children looking out all the windows of their home.

The honeymoon period ended quickly. Eliza began feeling alone and not an active part of her husband's life. Even though her husband was self-employed and worked at home all the time, they seldom talked during the weekday, and he often took his dinner in his office. Still Eliza, above all, felt grateful to be loved and safe in her home.

Eliza enjoyed a happy career from 1985 to 1994. She had an awesome boss and co-workers, and received an award for unwavering dedication to her sales team. Other staff outside of her department had trouble embracing Eliza's direct method of communication. Others did not understand Eliza's impatience with others not taking work seriously. Many times, Eliza felt misunderstood by many employees at her place of work. Her job became so stressful at times that Eliza just sat alone in her bedroom looking out the window after a day's work. Eliza continued with her position for eight years, until she became pregnant with her first child.

At this time in her life, Eliza's point of view immediately changed to a one-track plan – being the best Mother she could be. She knew these high expectations would come with significant coping struggles and an unhealthy amount of sleep deprivation. She was counting on support from her in-laws and most of all her husband and sister.

How much sleep is enough...and why?

- Among the middle-aged and older adult population, less than 6 hours sleep at night-time may be associated with depressive symptoms, but the symptoms can be improved with longer daytime naps.
- Less than 5 hours of sleep/night may increase the risk of diabetes by 58% and obesity by 48%, in comparison to 7–8 hours of sleep/night.
- Less than 6 hours of sleep/night may increase the prevalence of hypertension by 66%.
- During night-time sleep, blood pressure reduces by 10–20%. When this reduction is absent due to lack of sleep, the risk of resistant hypertension and cardiovascular mortality increases.
- Those with less optimal night-time sleep have significantly higher odds for diabetes, obesity, and various heart diseases.
- Those with a sleep duration shorter or longer than 7–8 hours/night and highly fragmented sleep may have significantly higher odds of high BMI and obesity.

(Zhu et al, 2021)

A UK Biobank study of sleep as a specific risk factor for poor metabolic and mental health (84,404 Participants); by far the largest UK accelerometry cohort to study sleep duration as a specific risk factor of metabolic and mental health.

Between age 26 and 35, Eliza drastically changed how she spent her free time to complement her role as wife and member of her in-law household. Her coping skills instead became enjoyable options.

- Dedicating many hours a day to practicing classical piano,

- Collecting and cooking many interesting recipes for her new family,

- Attending family gatherings with her in-laws,

- Going to bed early to have time alone with her thoughts,

- Enjoying only having to work one job with every evening free, and

- Joining the local gym.

DISCUSSION

It is amazing how a human being can seamlessly adjust to major life-changing situations. As easy as 123, one bright, blossoming career is changed into one far better and more important than anything accomplished before. Mothers are and always will be key to the backbone of society. It doesn't matter what wars are going on or what Mother Nature is cooking up. Mothers steadfastly keep their footing and remain focused on the care of their children and safety at home. There's no need for a plan B; Mothers make sure plan A is always the best possible scenario for their family.

The job title of "Mother" remains undervalued even in today's modern society (Crittenden, 2002). The monetary value of a Mother's unpaid workload has never been measured and is, therefore, "not counted towards a country's gross domestic product" (Dean et al, 2022). It is assumed a Mother does her work out of love deep in her heart, allowing it to flow into all aspects of life. A Mother's mental load is easily doubled or more, all out of the sight of others and quietly adopted as part of the job of being a full-time mom (Edgley, 2021).

PHASE FIVE – ACCELERATION OF

EVERYTHING

AGE 35 TO 45 – DIVING HEADFIRST INTO

MOTHERHOOD

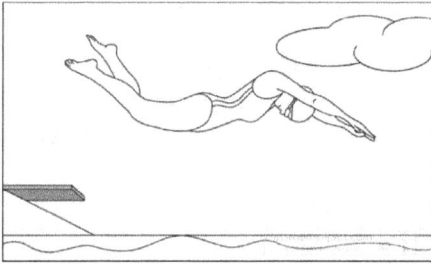

In 1993 at age 35 Eliza gave birth to a beautiful, healthy 7-pound baby girl. Within 6 weeks of giving birth, Eliza became pregnant with her second child. This pregnancy was at very high risk of hydrops fetalis (Younge et al, 2023). Eliza endured numerous blood and amniocentesis tests until the baby was old enough for birth induction. In 1994, eleven months later, her second beautiful daughter was born at 7.6 pounds with no health problems. Eliza and her husband were clearly advised by the pediatrician to not have any more children because of the high risks for baby.

Eliza catapulted straight into Motherhood. Now is the time Eliza wished for six arms like the "Silver Maiden" in the 1940 movie, "Thief of Bagdad." Every day consisted of continuous diaper changing, preparing formula, washing bottles, doing laundry and so on. Very soon into Motherhood Eliza knew sleep deprivation. She was so exhausted that standing most of the day was the only option. Sitting for just a few minutes meant nodding off and not watching her children properly. There was only one bad event when Eliza forgot she was sterilizing the bottle nipples in boiling water; all the water evaporated, and smoke came from the pan as the nipples melted.

Thief of Bagdad, 1940, film clip of the "Silver Maiden."   https://www.youtube.com/watch?v=nidEcn4pjqU

Support was offered by her in-laws only when it was convenient for them, seldom when Eliza desperately needed to rest. She often felt judged as an incompetent Mother. More than once, her Mother-in-law took her baby directly out of Eliza's arms without asking if that was okay. When Eliza did say something, Mother-in-law's response was usually "tough." Eliza was watched closely every single morning during baby's bath time. If either of the girls cried for any length of time, up came the in-laws from below to see what's wrong. These impromptu visits were always accompanied with suggestions, leaving Eliza feeling twisted.

In 1997, Eliza and her husband purchased a separate single-family home about a two-hour drive from family. This felt freeing for Eliza to Mother her children her way without daily comments. The only negative of being farther away was that the children missed their grandparents. Visits normally occurred every two or three months, most notably on Easter and Thanksgiving holidays.

Eliza was always with her daughters watching over them carefully and doing her best to keep the house clean and her children happy. Eliza handled all the errands, cooking and housekeeping with no assistance. No one offered to buy groceries or cook the meals. Eliza's only break was when the girls napped maybe once a day. Her younger daughter often didn't seem to need naps, which meant no one napped on those days.

What is the value of a nap?

- Napping between the afternoon hours of 1 and 5 pm can improve cognitive performance, such as: addition, logical reasoning, reaction time, and symbol recognition.
- Napping may be beneficial for all types of memory – procedural, declarative, or short-term memory.
- Daytime napping has the benefits of relaxation, reduced fatigue and improved mood.
- Daytime nappers may have improved mental productivity, physical performance and it may help people cope with fatigue related to shiftwork.
- Time for cardiovascular recovery may be gained by napping along with reduction of psychological stress.
- To avoid sleep inertia (i.e., the period of feeling groggy upon awaking), naps should be short (20–30 min).

(Dutheil et al, 2021)

Gradually, Eliza noticed a high sensitivity to bright lights and loud sounds. Even her own voice felt unbearably loud. The reason behind this was never diagnosed. Eliza did research on her own and learned it is possible her brain is "highly sensitive" (Fehlmann et al, 2023). The research also stated patients with these symptoms are often misdiagnosed with autism. This was not the case for Eliza. There is no cure for 'sensitive brain syndrome.' Avoiding bright lights and loud sounds seemed like the best solution. Speaking softly helped reduce the severity but at a price. People often couldn't hear Eliza, necessitating repetition which was the last thing Eliza wanted to do.

What does it mean to have a highly sensitive brain?

- "Differences in sensitivity are explained by both genetic (47%) and environmental factors (53%), such as family, work, school, culture, etc."
- "Not shy. On the alert."
- Deeper conscious and subconscious processing.
- Details about the environment and interactions with others are processed more deeply.
- Heightened empathy and emotional responsiveness
- Easily over stimulated or overwhelmed

(Fehlmann et al, 2023)

Phase Five – Acceleration of Everything

When Eliza's daughters were ages 2 and 3, her mental capacity to cope reached the point of screaming. Eliza was in the bathroom helping the girls take a bath and get dressed for bed. It was the end of a very long day being completely alone with the girls and Eliza was exhausted. She was sincerely ready for the girls to get in bed so dad could start their evening reading ritual. The girls always seemed to have a lot of energy directly after dinner and, on this particular evening, they were both feeling wound up tight and refusing to cooperate. Eliza called dad up to take over. She then went to the master bedroom and screamed for the first time.

Meditation Done *Your* Way

Meditation didn't come easy for Eliza. During her labor with her first daughter, she tried concentrating on the cover of a magazine, retracing the letters of the word 'one' over and over again in her head. She dutifully did the shallow short breathing with firm focus. After several tries, Eliza flung the magazine across the room and told her husband, "This isn't working!"

When Eliza's children were both very young, she desperately tried a variety of meditation methods, also without success.

Now at age 62, Eliza grasped meditation by laying still on her back in bed and giving all her focus to inhaling and exhaling. This helps Eliza quiet her mind and fall sleep more quickly.

Eliza had trouble getting through even just one day without yelling at the girls about something. She consulted with their family physician who assured Eliza she was not alone, sharing that she too did a lot of yelling when her children were young. During one visit with her brother, David, Eliza shared her frustration with always feeling like she was on the verge of yelling. David validated her feeling, sharing that he often feels the same way even though he is not caring for young children.

The girls went to preschool followed by kindergarten and first grade at a St. Mary's Catholic school in town. Feeling terribly constricted by Catholic School rules and pressured to get both girls baptized as soon as possible, Eliza and her husband elected to begin homeschooling their children starting grade 2.

Eliza tried working part time as a medical transcriptionist at home while home-schooling their children. This lasted a short while until her husband felt it would be a great idea for both parents to become licensed real estate agents. This did quickly happen with Eliza working every chance she had and her husband continuing his "bread winner" full time job, helping with real estate tasks as time allowed. The children were educated during the day by mom and in the evening by their dad. Mom spent every free minute making real estate calls and lining up appointments for the weekend. Eliza had to be ready in a moment's notice to change direction and focus. One minute mom duties mandated, and the next Eliza turned completely around to helping clients, back and forth all day. This mental load (Dean et al, 2022) was far more than Eliza could handle.

This constant responsibility and pressure made Eliza feel heavy, like the space above her was closing in. Eliza searched earnestly for a mother's helper and was able to hire a high school girl who lived nearby. This gave Eliza a helpful few hours per week break. Other babysitters came and went with no one being the perfect fit. Once, each of the girls spent a weekend at their grandparents. On one other occasion, Eliza's sister took the girls for the weekend. These are the only instances Eliza had a complete rest from Motherhood.

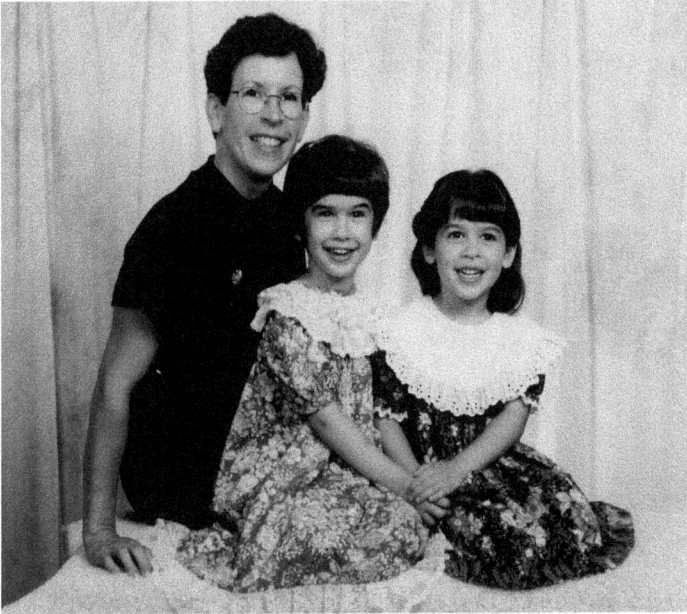

Eliza and her daughters

Next came a huge speed bump. Eliza's husband, the breadwinner, was suddenly laid off. Despite repeated attempts to find replacement work at the same salary, the only available option was a job that was only one third of his previous salary. Eliza and her husband had to make some quick financial decisions. The best option at the time seemed to be to sell their home and move to Maine, closer to her husband's family. At this time in their marriage, Eliza freely accepted her husband's decisions about what was best for their family unit.

The move to Maine couldn't have been more awful during the first two years there. Eliza's husband went from a 100% desk job to full blue collar carpenter work. Only a few months into this work, her husband herniated a disk in the lower back, completely incapacitating him for months. Many a day was spent with him bent over the side of the bed on his knees reeling in pain, with their two young children in the background clearly noticing all of it. During the next twelve months, Eliza put the family on State health coverage and food stamps. She also had to start working a full-time job at minimum wage. The children stayed home with dad while Eliza did everything else. Their financial situation was poor, down at one point to $200 cash on hand. An anonymous donation came from her husband's family and Eliza's brother, David, sent them a $1000 gift. This helped them keep warm and put food on the table.

By age 45, Eliza adapted her coping skills and daily tasks to align with being an attentive, on-demand Mother and stable full time social worker for a community non-profit:

- Isolation at the end of the day in her bedroom away from demands and questions,

- Surrounding herself with books, literally bookshelves on every wall with the bed in the middle of the room,

- Jogging outdoors or speed walking,

- Relaxing on the sofa with her canine buddy, Benny the beagle, leaning on her shoulder,

- Relaxing in the tub of hot water every evening while her husband read to the children, and

- Speaking softly and avoiding raising her voice as much as possible.

DISCUSSION

What makes a person reach the point of screaming? "Mental load is the combination of the cognitive labor of family life – the thinking, planning, scheduling and organizing of family members and the emotional labor associated with this work, including the feelings of caring and being responsible for family members but also the emotional impact of this work." (Dean et al, 2022). The "mental load" of Motherhood is often not visible to others, even those who live under the same roof. People give the most immediate attention to their own thoughts and tasks at hand. Normally, if there isn't a ruckus, there's no notice of how anyone in the household is coping. In this story we have Eliza, a young stay-at-home Mother, with little support and an unfathomable mental load. Eliza still doesn't yet know she has a mental illness, so all her struggles and mental anguish are just swallowed, as if nothing extraordinary is happening.

There are no boundaries (Dean, Churchill, Ruppanner, 2022) to Motherhood responsibilities, especially from the mother's point of view. Mothers do whatever needs to be done to keep their family safe, warm and nourished. What people see from the outside looking in is a family having dinner together. No one thinks about who bought the food, cooked the meal or cleaned up afterward. None of the daily duties to keep the laundry done, pantry stocked, house clean, and kids driven to sports events or medical appointments happen magically. It is assumed Mothers automatically take on these responsibilities. Let's not forget being up all night with sick children and holding the vomit bucket! So where does the time and guilt-free energy come from for Mothers to tend to their own needs? We aren't talking about a trip to the beauty salon or a massage at the spa; this is about time needed to stay physically and psychologically healthy. On top of that and most importantly, how does time for a mental illness fit in between everything else? It doesn't. Mothers just keep doing what they're supposed to do in the eyes of the public but also deep within their own conscience.

The emotion and care connected with those we love deeply is never complete because it is constant (Dean et al, 2022). Mothers cannot hire someone to handle monitoring their children's emotional well-being. A Mother's love is life-long. The well-being of her children is on display for everyone to see. This is constant pressure to "get it right" all the time without fail. This is a job unlike any other; there's no clocking in/out and everyone feels free to render opinions. A "regular" paid job is so much easier; the only concerning opinions are those of the employer (Crittenden, 2002).

Eliza is a survivor of life-long psychological and physical abuse – from her parents, siblings, school peers, neighborhood children and employers. Eliza was created from a lustful encounter between adults. Her parents made no sacrifices for their children. The beauty of having a close, loving family unit was not present in her home. Eliza grew up lonely with no true understanding of the importance of family, *until* she created her own family unit.

Eliza broke the bad parenting cycle within her family history. Together with her husband of 40 years, they raised two daughters. No abuse of any kind; just an abundance of love and making their children feel needed and wanted. Lust had nothing to do with it. Today they live within a 20-minute drive of their children.

What's all the huff and puff about breathing?

"Your breath is the only system in your body that is both automatic *and* under your control. Breathing is the bridge between mind and body. When you change your breath, you change your nervous system back to a calm state."

Here's a sampling of breathing practices that can be used anytime, anywhere for anxiety and stress relief.

- Box Breathing – inhale to a count of 4, hold to 4, exhale to 4, hold to 4. Repeat 4 times.
- 4-7-8 Breathing – inhale to a count of 4, hold to 7, exhale to 8
- Sigh It Out – inhale gently, then exhale through your mouth with a full-body sigh.
- Hand on Heart Breath – place your hand over your heart. Breathe slowly and say, "I've got me."

(Resilience Within, 2025)

PHASE SIX – THE DARKEST RIDE

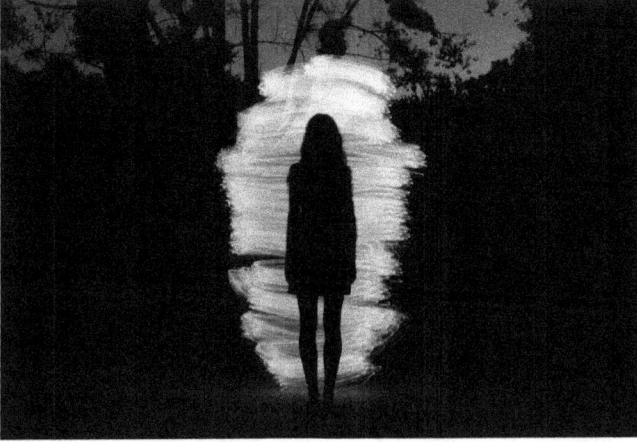

freepick.com 1

The next 15 years would be the most emotionally draining of Eliza's life. There were continuous dips and curves in the road taking Eliza on an exasperating ride. Eliza's resilience to continue plugging along and keep her family safe, fed and warm was her spark to repeatedly get back up and keep moving forward. It was her immediate family unit's heavy dependence on her that helped Eliza keep her head up.

AGE 45 TO 60 – CHAOS AND CHANGE

Eliza's husband connected to what seemed to be a good primary care doctor who prescribed a mix of opioids for pain relief. The dosage kept increasing each month for the next ten years. Next Ambien was added to help with sleep. Eliza witnessed and helped her husband after 2nd degree burns on his hands from leaning on a boiling hot wood stove while in a sleeping stupor from Ambien. The lingering sleepy after-effects of this drug caused her husband to get in two totaled car accidents. It was later publicized that Ambien did not completely leave the system of patients after a night's sleep. Eliza's family endured a lawsuit for each accident which dragged on for two years.

Eliza's husband managed to obtain a solid full-time job despite his back pain and opioid use. Financially things were settled for her family. Eliza started a full-time job as a social worker for the elderly and disabled adult population. The family moved to a big house on several acres and lived there from 2005 until 2019. Here their daughters grew up and went through the tumultuous teenage years. Eliza handled all day-to-day household tasks in addition to working full-time and providing transportation to/from school and events for the girls.

Eliza's daily workday routine consisted of waiting for the girls to get ready for school, driving them there and then heading off to her job. She ate lunch at her desk every workday because she needed to spend that hour picking up the girls from school, driving them home and coming back to finish her workday. Every single school morning, Eliza was late to work because her oldest daughter could not get ready on time. Eliza was at high risk of losing her job and was "talked to" several times by her boss. She felt like she was spiraling out of control.

Eliza, now age 47, connected with a primary care physician (PCP) who gave her first diagnosis of clinical depression and anxiety (American Psychiatric

Association, DSM-5, 2013). Eliza began taking anti-depressants and started to feel better, less anxious. Eliza was 10 minutes late for one of her regular appointments with her PCP and was told she could not be seen and had to reschedule. On this day in particular, Eliza desperately needed to be seen. The PCP staff didn't know Eliza's oldest daughter that morning told her mom she hated her, all because mom would not go back home so her daughter could put on deodorant. Eliza was late to her doctor appointment because of this. That day, after Eliza dropped the girls at school, she just sat in the parking lot trying to process what was said. She really needed to talk with *someone*. The front office medical staff refused to listen. Eliza had to just keep on going about her regular work and family tasks no matter how sad she felt.

Eliza started to experience formication, the delusional sensation of bugs crawling under her skin, especially down the back of her neck (Coetzee et al,

2022). Her PCP just gave her a head nod and sad expression when Eliza brought it up at a medical appointment. No suggestions were given for relief. This was tormenting for Eliza who often held her hand to the back of her neck for relief. Employees at work started to notice and inquire. To keep face, Eliza told them her neck was painful.

In 2012 both of Eliza's daughters went off to college. Eliza, at age 47, took advantage of her new learned experience of applying to college and getting financial aid. From 2012 to 2017 Eliza went back to college and finished her undergraduate degree. This was a positive experience for Eliza because she was doing this *just* for herself; time spent studying felt therapeutic and, at times, invigorating. Eliza kept working full time and moved through college at a very quick pace. She graduated magna cum laude with a grade point average of 3.97.

Between 2012 and 2017, Eliza changed primary care physicians (PCP) three more times and went through three psychologists. None were a good fit, especially when the psychologists each time started to talk about themselves during the sessions. Two of the PCPs just kept pumping her full of meds that did not help with depression or anxiety but did cause a 20-pound weight gain. During this same time period, Eliza landed in the Emergency Room (ER) several times with stress-related ailments and difficulty sleeping. She was prescribed Ambien and took it only once just before bedtime. The next morning, she awoke to her husband asking her to let him take her back to the ER. Eliza remembered nothing about the night's events – vomiting, laying on the floor, talking incoherently. The ER doctor believed this was entirely caused by Ambien and Eliza's complete exhaustion. She was advised to take a month off from work and just rest. Eliza would have jumped at that idea but couldn't because she was a Mother of two teenage children and on duty 24/7. Eliza made the poor choice to just keep going as she was – working fulltime, driving the girls everywhere needed, managing the household budget, cooking, cleaning, etc.

In August of 2012, Eliza's brother, David, committed suicide. For a long time, David suffered from war PTSD and deep depression (Levi-Belz et al, 2022). He was on and off medications all his post-war life. He survived triple bypass surgery and was called a role model patient for his quick recovery. David's PCP was associated with the Veterans Administration. David was seen about a mark on his shoulder and told it was nothing consequential by a VA PCP. One year later, David was diagnosed with advanced melanoma and subject to urgent surgery. He did not recover well. Eliza believed this post-op pain sent him over the edge. David opened his weapons safe and laid the weapons on his bed sheets. He chose a weapon, loaded it, held the pistol to his left ear and fired. A few days before his suicide, David talked to everyone important in his life and said, "I love you." For years to follow, Eliza had flash backs about her brother. Just something as simple as remembering he loved to eat pistachio nuts, would trigger the memory of his suicide.

In 2015, Eliza became very sick with a high fever and severe lung congestion. Her current PCP just kept telling Eliza that her lung x-ray was clean. Lab work was mostly normal. Eliza requested to be referred to a pulmonologist who, after two bouts of antibiotics, was able to help Eliza's lungs heal. Eliza requested the pulmonologist's suggestion for a good PCP. She was referred to an excellent one who took good care of Eliza until 2020. This PCP reached the point with a high patient panel that she often was not available to see her primary patients for a sick appointment. Sometimes even the annual exams had to be rescheduled. After much searching, Eliza located a new PCP with a different practice much closer to home. Because she was a new PCP to that practice, she was able to take on new patients. This led to an excellent connection with a counselor who, to this day, has been incredibly helpful to Eliza. Both of these medical professionals have had a significant impact in helping Eliza stay off the edges of her mental illness.

Eliza had her first visual hallucination in the early morning hours of her 60th birthday. It is not uncommon for her to visit the bathroom several times every evening. This one time, while she was sitting there half asleep, she looked down at the rug and everything was moving. The rug fibers turned into creepy crawly worm-like creatures that were the same color of the rug. The entire floor looked like it was moving. Eliza really wasn't sure if it was real or not, so she put her foot down on the rug to see if she could feel them. She could not. Eliza looked over to the doorway and there sat her cat looking down at the rug. She wondered if the cat could see them. Eliza turned the lights on and could see it was visual fiction.

She checked her pupils and could see they were not dilated. Eliza carried this hallucination in her mind for several days. Eliza hoped that this wasn't a sign she was slowly losing her mind. She never shared this with anyone for fear of judgment.

Now that the children were legally adults and mostly living on their own, Eliza and her husband decided to sell their home and move to a location closer to her husband's family. This move was a huge undertaking because her husband accumulated so much "stuff" that every part of their 4,000 square foot house was full. In the fall of 2019, their house sold, and Eliza's family moved into a temporary small house while they searched to buy a new home closer to family.

As soon as COVID hit, Eliza and her husband were permitted to work full time from home. This was a huge positive change to their family. The stress of commuting a long distance to work was removed from the daily picture. It is at this time that Eliza's husband decided to detox from opioids cold turkey 100% on his own. His PCP did not inform the family, "because he felt certain this approach was safe in that he had suggested this type of detox to former patients."

The next five days were the scariest for Eliza and her daughters. Her husband's doctor would not speak directly to Eliza because of breaching patient/doctor confidentiality. It wasn't until after Eliza threatened a law suit did his PCP returned her call. His PCP immediately dropped her husband as a patient. Eliza was able to find another practice to take him in as a patient. Her husband did successfully survive detox and has not touched a drop of opioids since that time. It took many months but eventually Eliza felt the man she married all those years ago had returned to her.

In 2020, soon after COVID hit, they moved into a permanent home within just a few miles of family. Eliza burned out from her social work job and switched to a job with significantly less stress.

By age 60, Eliza settled nicely into her daily routine and coping skills:

- Daily segments of time away from everyone with complete silence,

- Religiously taking her anti-depressant medication,

- Regular scalp, shoulder and back massages,

- Moving at a much slower pace, reducing multitasking,

- Walking outside as much as possible,

- Playing classical piano,

- Listening to music, and

- Slow, steady deep breathing.

The State of Mental Health in America

- "23.08% of adults experienced a mental illness in the past year, equivalent to nearly 60 million Americans. Of this group, 5.86% experienced a severe mental illness, approximately 3.5 million.

- As of March 2024, over 122 million people lived in a mental health workforce shortage area, and only 27% of the mental health needs in these areas were being met by mental health providers.

- 2022 Had the highest number of deaths by suicide ever recorded in America."

(Reinert et al, 2024)

DISCUSSION

The world is in a humanitarian crisis (Troup, 2021). Barriers continue to multiply. Facilitators are needed to break down barriers and lead in the reconstruction of better care (Troup, 2021). The biggest challenge is keeping up with the rapidly increasing rate of mental disorder diagnoses (GBD 2019 Mental Disorders Collaborators, 2022).

Half of the world's population will develop a mental health disorder by age 75. Typically, the first symptoms of mental illness begin before age 21. The three most common mental illnesses are depression, anxiety and post-traumatic stress syndrome (McGrath, 2023). For decades, mental health services and treatment have been grossly insufficient to respond to the need. (Troup, 2021 & GBD, 2019).

"Definitions of mental illnesses have changed over the last half-century. Mental illness refers to conditions that affect cognition, emotion, and behavior…"

(Manderscheid et all, 2010). The lifelong daily challenges for someone with a mental illness remain undervalued and misunderstood. Life's journey is challenging even to the most intelligent and financially solvent person. Multiply those challenges ten-fold for someone with a mental illness.

Eliza's experiences with medical care have left her believing the medical system is broken (Geyman, 2021). There has been significant research about person-centered care and coordinated patient care across the disciplines (Fulmer et al, 2021). This only works if medical staff and insurance companies are in sync with allocating enough time and money to sufficiently care for patients.

In addition, many health practices hold medical staff to goals through Key Performance Indicators (KPIs) (Sreedharan et al, 2024). This only works if the KPIs are aligned with patient care. Eliza worked at a major medical facility in Maine that required mandatory attendance at weekly staff meetings to review KPIs and share progress toward reaching them. Every department in this medical facility of more than 15,000 employees was required to attend this virtual meeting every Monday. The KPIs were largely related to ongoing projects and not directly to patient care. Some were more focused on reaching more patients to justify the number of paid staff on the budget. Where do the patients fall in the priority list?

Eliza received her first "official" diagnosis at the age of 47 – chronic anxiety and clinical depression. Before this time, she had no idea what was going on with her head. The symptoms of these diagnoses kept pushing her back to bed. Sleep and complete silence continue to be her escape. Patients should not have to wait all those years for answers.

Fear of being "blue papered" (i.e., involuntarily admitted to a psych ward) loomed whenever Eliza shared any of her mental illness symptoms. Patients dare not discuss these experiences with family or friends. What would they think of us? Eliza did not tell anyone about her hallucination. She seldom discussed her mental health with anyone. Eliza is sharing her symptoms now with readers, hoping there must be a distant kindred spirit out there.

What caused Eliza's hallucination? Did she have too much sugar the day before or was this just an anomaly in her brain this one time? Maybe she has had other hallucinations, but this is the only one in memory. How can patients know the true reasons behind what they feel, see and do? It is impossible to solve this puzzle and herein lies the consistent frustration in understanding mental health. While it may be said that a patient knows her body better than anyone else, patients struggle just like medical professionals to unravel the mystery of brain behavior. The big difference between patients and medical professionals when it comes to these experiences is the patients are *affected* while the professionals continue to *ponder*.

Hallucinations

- "Hallucinations defined as the perception of an object or event (in any of the 5 senses), in the absence of an external stimulus, are experienced by patients with conditions that span several fields (e.g., psychiatry, neurology, and ophthalmology)."
- There are six different types of hallucinations, each with multiple subcategories (i.e., auditory, visual, olfactory, gustatory, somatic and tactile).
- "Despite more than 20 years of clinical and experimental research, it remains unclear how hallucinations occur only in some people and only at some times."
- Eliza had only one hallucinogenic visual episode, thus did not pursue further evaluation.
- Of the more than 20 possible causes of hallucinations, Eliza believes her hallucination was probably caused by sleep deprivation and intense emotional experiences.

(Ali et al, 2011) – (Collerton et al, 2023) – (Teeple et al, 2009)

PHASE SEVEN – COASTING FREEFORM

AGE 60 TO PRESENT – A WHOLE

NEW POINT OF VIEW

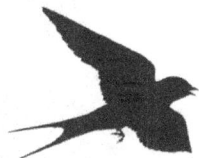

The manual brake is pulled. No more clenched hands or hairpin curves. Eliza's rollercoaster ride is over. The remaining years of her life are free time for Eliza to enjoy coasting, with the security of a toolbox by her side full of coping strategies and many lessons learned. No time schedule and free from judgment. The only remaining obligations are those Eliza chooses to keep.

Eliza's love and dedication to her daughters never withered. So strong is the bond between Mother and child, especially daughters. Even the most heated arguments or harshest words will not change a Mother's love for her children.

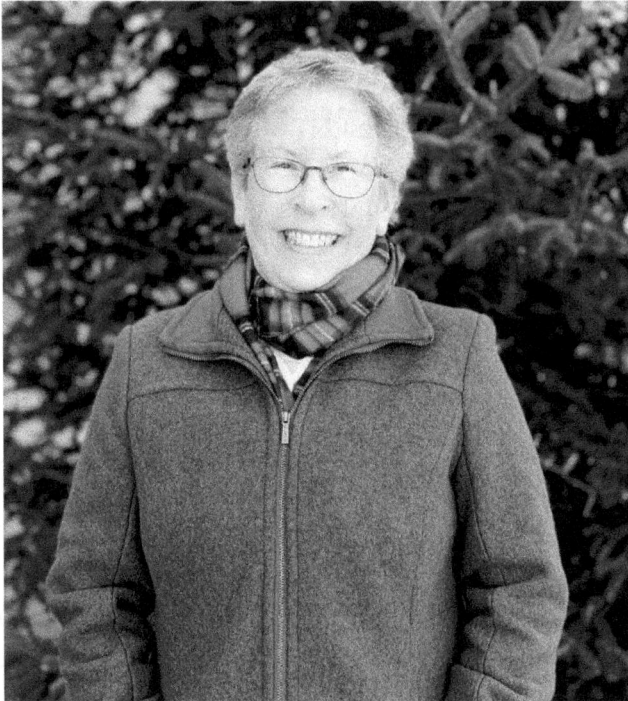

Eliza age 60

COVID in 2020 was more freeing than challenging for Eliza. She liked wearing a mask because she didn't have to walk around with a fake smile. So many people had wrinkled brows just like Eliza's, but for very different reasons. The public in general were emotionally distressed because COVID brought about concerns they've never had to face. Mental illness cases soared during COVID. For Eliza, this was old hat.

COVID allowed Eliza to be secluded and absent from many public events without judgment.

Still to this day Eliza suffers from symptoms of formication (i.e., feeling as if imaginary bugs are crawling under the skin). Now the formication is also on her forehead in addition to the back of her neck. This is very distracting especially when trying to fall asleep. There is no cure.

Eliza retired from all full-time work at age 62. Eliza's lost income forced Eliza and her husband to make substantial financial changes. Eliza handled the household budget and monitored all spending. She became the 'budget bitch,' often calling her husband out for large cumulative music purchases. Eliza also had to step back from buying without looking at the prices. Her husband was a good provider allowing Eliza the freedom to put whatever she liked in the grocery cart every week. Both of them had habits that needed to stop.

In March of 2022, Eliza completed the paperwork for student debt relief from Nelnet.com. With Eliza's PCP's assistance, her mental health diagnoses and screenings for depression and anxiety scored high enough to make her eligible for total student debt forgiveness, including the Parent Plus loans she had taken out for her daughters. The relief felt after receiving written notification seemed surreal. The enormous financial weight was lifted. Now Eliza's only task was to continue living a full life.

Eliza and her husband now had an empty nest, with both daughters living independently but nearby. The house felt so empty. With a lot of time on her hands and a need to feel useful, at age 62, Eliza began documenting her lifelong journey with mental illness. Eliza found writing about her own mental illness to be an enormous challenge. She had to remember and constantly revisit every detail of the abuse and neglect. Her goal in sharing this story is to leave readers feeling validated and less alone. Each writing session left Eliza feeling totally beaten down. The writing sessions had to be short enough to get through the content before hitting bottom again. Walking away from each writing session recreated her sadness and loneliness, often taking weeks for Eliza to feel strong enough to continue.

Throughout her life, Eliza has only seen one psychiatrist for medication adjustment. Eliza has been through five psychologists and nine primary care practitioners. Today, Eliza at age 67 is receiving excellent consultation and care from a PCP only ten minutes from home.

During her lifetime, Eliza held 31 different jobs and changed living residences 21 times, living between the states of Maine and Virginia. The lesson learned is that one job or living quarters really isn't any better than the other. Eliza now realizes that she was missing companionship and unconditional love. Her forty years of marriage and two children filled in those blanks beautifully!

Eliza's anxiety is still not well-controlled today by her medications. It's as if her worries are floating freeform. The worries easily shift from a genuine ongoing stressful situation to a possible 'future' situation that may arise. Eliza cannot rationalize her worries away. It doesn't help to hear someone say, "you don't have any control over the future" or "why think of such sad possibilities?" Anxiety is driven by emotions not logic. When anxiety rears its ugly head, Eliza opens her toolbox and pulls from it what has worked to calm thoughts down in the past.

The Anxiety Reset

For persistent anxiety and worry caused by stress, genetics or brain chemistry, try any of these daily rituals to "rewire" your mind and body back to a calm state. Doing this as a repetitive routine is best.

- 5-4-3-2-1 Senses Scan – Name 5 things you can see, 4 you can touch, 3 you can hear, 2 you can smell and 1 you taste.
- Feel Your Feet – Stand or sit. Focus all attention on the soles of your feet. Press them down.
- Anchor Object – Hold a familiar object and describe it silently – texture, temperature, weight.
- Name the Moment – Say: "This is anxiety. I'm feeling it, not becoming it."

(Jantz et al, 2021 & Resilience Within, 2025)

Eliza has finally come home to a peaceful life setting she has created over the years. She describes her peace as the sensation of flowing through each day with no stress. Her point of view has become less critical and more forgiving of the missteps of others.

At this point in Eliza's life, she has nailed down her most useful coping skills. She continues with her daily routines to maintain calmness, which include one or more of the following as often as needed:

- Daily time for self-reflection,

- Isolation in her bedroom away from voices and noise to focus on the importance of slow, deep breathing,

- Cracking the window open near her bed to hear the birds and feel a wonderful puff of air on her face,

- Silencing all electric notifications,

- Listening to classical music,

- Reading physical books, not Kindle or online,

- Speaking as softly as possible,

- Walking outside as much as possible,

- Sitting outside during the first snow of the season and embracing the soft sound of snowflakes landing on the ground,

- Having a cup of tea and listening to Maine Public Radio,

- Enjoying the freeform feeling of exercising in the local YMCA therapy pool; no pain but plenty gained,

- Frequent naps, as often as she liked, with no hesitation or feelings of guilt,

- Eating less cottage cheese and more ice cream, sometimes too often (Bombeck, 2003). Stopped focusing on possible weight gain,

- Enjoying the solitude of writing and researching,

- Learning to savor complete quiet in her bedroom, and

- Realizing that having less to do and being comfortable alone can feel like so much more than it sounds to others.

DISCUSSION

Eliza created her own list of coping mechanisms as she went through life. Her list changed often to handle health changes, marital struggles, and maturing children. These coping strategies kept Eliza from plunging off the deep end with her emotions. Eliza's dedication to Motherhood and keeping her family unit safe kept her off the edge many times.

Eliza refused to let a diagnosis get in the way of having a wonderfully meaningful life. She took a step back to get a running start and leap right over any barriers. Eliza repeated this action every time that diagnosis reared its ugly head or the unkind loud words of someone echoed in her head.

Eliza never accepted negative connotations from family, peers, employers, and the general public. Her medical illness diagnosis *did not* define her. In fact, upon deep reflection, Eliza believes her diagnosis has made her *more* observant of situations and people. Her mental illness made Eliza keenly aware of the power of words and opinions. Eliza developed good communications skills, not from a mentor, but from the bad example of others. She immediately learned what *not to* do or say when interacting with people, especially during the first contact.

Words are powerful. Eliza listened to her words and dreams. She extended her arms, stretched, and reached to the highest edge of conscious thought. Eliza kept wanting for something better. To this day she continues to identify and firmly hold onto moments in life that give her joy and hope.

Benefits of Aquatic Exercise

- Exercise in an aquatic environment may provide a significant reduction in abdominal fat.
- Aquatic exercise programs may have positive effects on functional fitness, mainly related to upper- and lower-limb strength.
- Aquatic exercise programs also tend to have a positive impact on agility and dynamic balance in older people.
- Positive improvements in cognitive function as a result of intervention with aquatic exercise in all exercise groups have been recognized.
- Weight-bearing activities in the water are much easier and the risk of falling in the elderly is less.
- Aquatic exercise with continuous intensity improves mental health (by reducing depression, anxiety, and stress)

  (Farinha et al, 2021) and (Silva et al, 2022)

ELIZA'S FAVORITE CHOICES FOR RESEARCH AND LEARNING.

1. Centers for Disease Control and Mental Health. https://www.cdc.gov/mental-health/caring/index.html

2. Depression and Bipolar Support Alliance https://www.dbsalliance.org/education/

3. Google Scholar, peer reviewed, within the last 5 years. https://scholar.google.com/

4. Life Stance Online Therapy & Psychiatry Appointments. https://lifestance.com/

5. Mental Health America https://mhanational.org/

6. National Alliance on Mental Illness (NAMI) https://www.nami.org/

7. National Council for Mental Well Being https://www.thenationalcouncil.org/

8. National Institute of Mental Health https://www.nimh.nih.gov/health/find-help

9. Substance Abuse and Mental Health Services Administration https://www.samhsa.gov/

10. Your college/university library and database with free lifetime access for alumni

SUMMARY OF COPING SKILLS

Phase One – Birth to age 10
- Isolate in her bedroom or the playroom
- Speak very little and make minimal eye contact
- Seldom ask questions or make a request for anything
- Never enter her parent's bedroom or Father's office
- Always be obedient and honest, to avoid scolding

Phase Two – age 10 to 18
- Meditation through hours of piano playing
- Focused learning: books often opened on the table partnered with a pencil and notebook
- Watch television alone
- Minimal socialization with peers
- Seldom leave the house

Phase Three – age 18 to 26
- Work two jobs to eliminate financial stress
- Borrow the use of a piano from her second job site.
- Exercise as much as possible
- Focus on part time college courses
- Seldom socialize; solitary isolation
- Spend leisure time laying on her bed listening to radio

Phase Four – age 26 to 35
- Practice classical piano often
- Collect and cook many interesting recipes
- Attend family gatherings with her in-laws
- Go to bed early to have time alone with her thoughts
- Enjoy only having to work one job with every evening free
- Join the local gym

Phase Five – age 35 to 45
- Isolate at the end of the day in bedroom
- Surround herself with books
- Jog or speed walk
- Relax on the sofa with her canine buddy
- Relax in tub of hot water every evening.
- Speak softly and avoid raising her voice

Phase Six – age 45 to 60
- Daily segments of time away from everyone with complete silence
- Religiously take anti-depressant medication
- Regular scalp, shoulder and back massages
- Move at a much slower pace, reducing multitasking
- Walk outside as much as possible
- Play classical piano
- Listen to music
- Slow, steady deep breathing

Phase Seven – age 60 to present day
- Daily time for self-reflection
- Isolate in bedroom away from noise
- Crack the window open near her bed to hear the birds and feel a puff of fresh air
- Silence electric gadgets
- Classical music
- Read
- Speak softly
- Walk outside
- Listen to the soft sound of snowflakes landing on the ground
- Enjoy a warm cup of tea
- Swim in YMCA therapy pool
- Frequent naps, no feelings of guilt
- Eat less cottage cheese and more ice cream (Bombeck, 2003).
- Enjoy the solitude of writing and researching
- Learn to savor complete quiet
- Realize that having less to do and being comfortable alone can feel like so much more than it sounds to others.

Epilogue

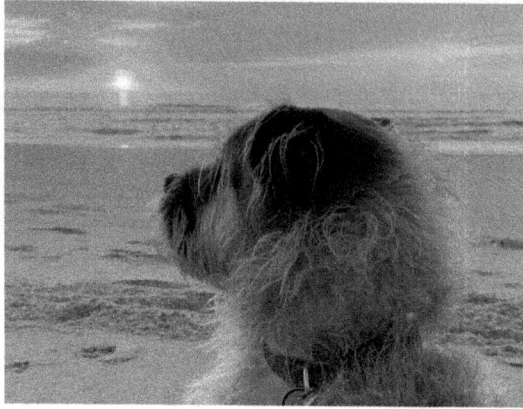

This is a true story. It is hard to believe these experiences are happening all the time, everywhere around the world. So many victims of mental illness remain painfully silent for fear of judgment. It is a daily challenge to find the best coping mechanism, sometimes just to get through the moment at hand. The consistent goal is to move away from the darkness and look for pieces of contentment. Fleeting moments of happiness are a bonus.

Deep thought is a powerful healer. These moments of self-reflection often bring forth something brilliant and meaningful, for both the writer and the reader. A diagnosis is the best first tool a patient can be given. Coping mechanisms offer an assortment of options for continuing forward.

Eliza is an ordinary woman, of normal IQ, possessing no particular gifted talents. She has a strong drive to make sense of happenings in her life. Eliza often stews over something because she needs an answer to the question, "why?" If an answer cannot be attained, Eliza walks away from the happening and strives to put it out of her mind. When confronted with something that feels uncomfortable, Eliza's first instinct is to get away from it as fast as possible. Back away now, think about later.

Thank you for reading her story. Even though mental illness is always lurking just beneath the surface, Eliza is optimistic that *anyone* can survive mental illness and have excellent quality of life. May this true story serve as inspiration, education and hope for a "good" life, despite any diagnoses.

References

REFERENCES

Ali, S., Patel, M., Avenido, J., Jabeen, S., Riley, W. J., & MBA, M. (2011). Hallucinations: Common features and causes. *Current Psychiatry, 10*(11), 22-29.

American Psychiatric Association, D. (2013). *Diagnostic and statistical manual of mental disorders: DSM-5* (5 ed.). Washington, D.C: American Psychiatric Association.

Arain, M., Hague, M., Johal, L., Mathur, P., Nel, W., Rais, A., & Sharma, S. (2013). Maturation of the adolscent brain. *Neuropsychiatric disease and treatment.*, 449-461.

Barchi, B. (2024). Family upbringing as a factor in the formation of children's emotional maturity. *Bulletin of National Defense, University of Ukraine, 2*(78), 18-22.

Best, O., & Ban, S. (2021). Adolescence: physical changes and neurological development. *British Journal of Nursing, 30*(5), 272-275.

Bombeck, E. (2003). *Eat less cottage cheese and more ice cream.* USA: Andrews McMeel Publishing.

Choudhury, S., Charman, T., & Blakemore, S. (2008). Development of the teenage brain. *Mind, Brain and Education*, 142-147.

References

Coetzee, S., Mahajan, C., & Franca, K. (2023). The diagnostic workup, screening, and treatment approaches for patients with delusional infestation. *Dermatology and Therapy, 13*(12), 2993-3006.

Collerton, D., Barnes, J., Diederich, N. J., Dudley, R., Friston, K., Goetz, C. G., & Weil, R. S. (2023). Understanding visual hallucinations: A new synthesis. *Neuroscience & biobehavioral reviews, 150,* 105208.

Crittenden, A. (2002). *The price of Motherhood: Why the most important job in the world is still the least valued.* New York, NY, USA: Metropolitan Books.

Dean, L., Churchill, B., & Ruppanner, L. (2022). The mental load: Building a deeper theoretical understanding of how cognitive and emotional labor overload women and Mothers. *Community, work & family, 25*(1), 31-29.

Dutheil, F., Danini, B., Bagheri, R., Fantini, M. L., Pereira, B., Moustafa, F., & Navel, V. (2021). Effects of a short daytime nap on the cognitive performance: a systematic review and meta-analysis. *International journal of environmental research and public health, 18*(19), 10212.

References

Farinha, C., Teixeira, A. M., Serrano, J., Santos, H., Campos, M. J., Oliveiros, B., & Ferreira, J. P. (2021). Impact of different aquatic exercise programs on body composition, functional fitness and cognitive function of non-institutionalized elderly adults: a randomized controlled trial. *International Journal of Environmental Research and Public Health, 18*(17), 8963.

Fehlmann, E., & Bresciani, S. (2023). The Highly Sensitive Brain. In E. N. Aron, Phd, *The Highly Sensitive Person: How to Thrive When the World Overwhelms You* (pp. 1-12). Switzerland: Associazione Kolours and Association High Sensitive Person Switzerland Lugano (Switzerland), 2023.

Fulmer, T., Reuben, D., Auerbach, J., Fick, D., Galambos, C., & Johnson, K. (2021). Actualizing Better Health and Health Care for Older Adults: Commentary describes six vital directions to improve the care and quality of life for all older Americans. *Health Affairs, 40*(2), 219-225.

GBD 2019 Mental Disorders Collaborators. (2022). Global, regional, and national burden of 12 mental disorders in 204 countries and territories. *The Lancet Psychiatry, 9*(2), 137-150.

Geyman, J. (2021). COVID-19 has revealed America's broken health care system: what can we learn? *International Journal of Health Sciences, 51*(2), 188-194.

References

Helbig, D. (2022). *Roller Coaster Terminology 101.* Retrieved February 17, 2024, from https://www.visitkingsisland.com/blog/2020/may/roller-coaster-terminology-101

Hristova, S. (2017). Blue Screen of Death: disrupting transparent windows, composite media, and the aesthetics of continuity. *Continuum, 31*(6), 833-843.

Huang, J. (2023). Impact of attachment style and school bullying. *SHS Web of Conferences - EDP Sciences, 180,* 03024.

Jantz, G. L., & Wall, K. (2021). *The Anxiety Reset.* Tyndale House Publishers, Inc.

Levi-Belz, Y., Shemesh, S., & Zerach, G. (2022). Moral Injury and suicide ideation among combat veterans. *Crisis Intervention and Suicide Prevention.*

Li, F., Luo, S., Mu, W., Li, Y., Ye, L., Zheng, X., & Chen, X. (2021). Effects of sources of social support and resilience on the mental health of different age groups during COVID-19 pandemic. *BMC Psychiatry, 21,* 1-14.

Maggi, S., Zaccaria, V., Breda, M., Romani, M., Aceti, F., Giacchetti, N., . . . Sogos, C. (2022). A narrative review about prosocial and antisocial behavior in childhood: The relationship with shame and moral development. *Children, 9*(10), 1556.

References

Manderscheid, R. W., Ryff, C. D., Freeman, E. J., McKnight-Eily, L. R., Dhingra, S., & Strine, T. W. (2010). Evolving definitions of mental illness and wellness. *Preventing chronic disease, 7*(1), A19.

McGrath, J., Al-Hamzawi, A., Alonso, J., Altwaijri, Y., Andrade, L., Bromet, E., & Zaslavsky, A. (2023). Age of onset and cumulative risk of mental disorders: a cross-national analysis of population surveys from 29 countries. *The Lancet Psychiatry, 10*(9), 668-681.

Merriam-Webster. (n.d.). Retrieved February 22, 2024, from https://www.merriam-webster.com/dictionary/

Reinert, M., Fritze, D., & Nguyen, T. (2024). *The state of mental health in America 2024.* Alexandra: Mental Health America. Retrieved from http://hdl.handle.net/10713/22688

Resilience , W. S. (2025). *Anxiety Reset: Body-Based Tools to feel Safe Again.* North Haven, CT, USA.

Selman, S. B., & Dilworth-Bart, J. E. (2024). Routines and child development: A systematic review. *Journal of Family Theory & Review, 16*(2), 272-328.

Silva, L. A., Menguer, L. D., Doyenart, R., Boeira, D., Milhomens, Y. P., Dieke, B., & Silveira, P. C. (2022). Effect of aquatic exercise on mental health, functional autonomy, and oxidative damages in diabetes elderly individuals. *International journal of environmental health research, 32*(9), 2098-2111.

Sreedharan, J., Subbarayalu, A. V., Kamalasanan, A., Albalawi, E., Krishna, G. G., Alahmari, A. D., &

References

MacDonald, J. (2024). Key performance indicators: a framework for allied healthcare educational institutions. *ClinicoEconomics and Outcomes Research*, 173-185.

Sultana, T., Ruiz-Casares, M., Iwo, R., Janus, M., & Nazif-Munoz, J. I. (2024). Maternal education and children home alone in 63 low- and middle-income countries. *Global Pediatric Health, 11*, 2333794X241258179.

Suniega, E. A., Krenek, L., & Stewart, G. (2022). Child abuse: approach and management. *American Family Physician, 105*(5), 521-528.

Susman, Susman, E., & Rogol, A. (2014). Puberty and psychological development. In R. M. Lerner, & L. Steinberg, *Handbook of adolescent psychology* (p. Chapter 2). Hoboken, NJ, USA: Wiley.

Syakhrani, A. W., & Aslan, A. (2024). The impact of informal family education on children's social and emotional skills. *Indonesian Journal of Education, 4*(2), 619-631.

Teeple, R. C., Caplan, J. P., & Stern, T. A. (2009). Visual halucinations: differential diagnosis and treatment. *Primary care companion to the journal of clinical psychiatry, 11*(1), 26.

References

Troup, J., Fuhr, D., Woodward, A., Sondorp, E., & Roberts, B. (2021). Barriers and facilitators for scaling up mental health and psychosocial support interventions in low-and mid-income countries for populations affected by humanitarian crises: a system review. *International Journal of Mental Health Systems, 15*, 1-14.

Wickramaratne, P. J., Yangchen, T., Lepow, L., Patra, B. G., Glicksburg, B., Talati, A., & Weissman, M. M. (n.d.). Social connectedness as a determinant of mental health. A scoping review. *PloS one, 17*(10), e0275004.

Younge, T., Ottolini, K. M., Al-Kouatly, H. B., & Berger, S. I. (2023). Hydrops fetalis: Incidence, Etiologies, management strategies and outcomes. *Research and Reports in Neonatology*, 81-92.

Zhu, G., Cassidy, S., Hiden, H., Woodman, S., Trenell, M., Gunn, D. A., & Anderson, K. N. (2021). Exploration of sleep as a specific risk factor for poor metabolic and mental health: A UK Biobank Study of 84,404 participants. *Nature and Science of Sleep*, 1903-1912.